Sensei Self Development

Mental Health Chronicles Series

Exploring Your Creativity

Sensei Paul David

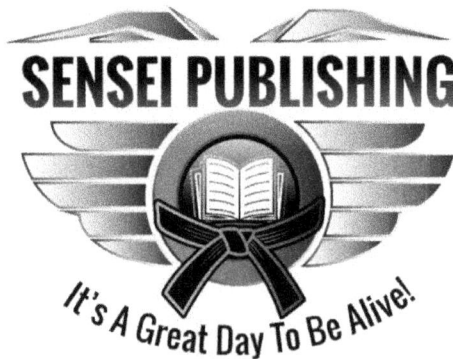

SENSEI PUBLISHING

It's A Great Day To Be Alive!

www.senseipublishing.com

@senseipublishing
senseipublishing

Get/Share Your FREE SSD Mental Health Chronicles at
www.senseiselfdevelopment.care

or

CLICK HERE

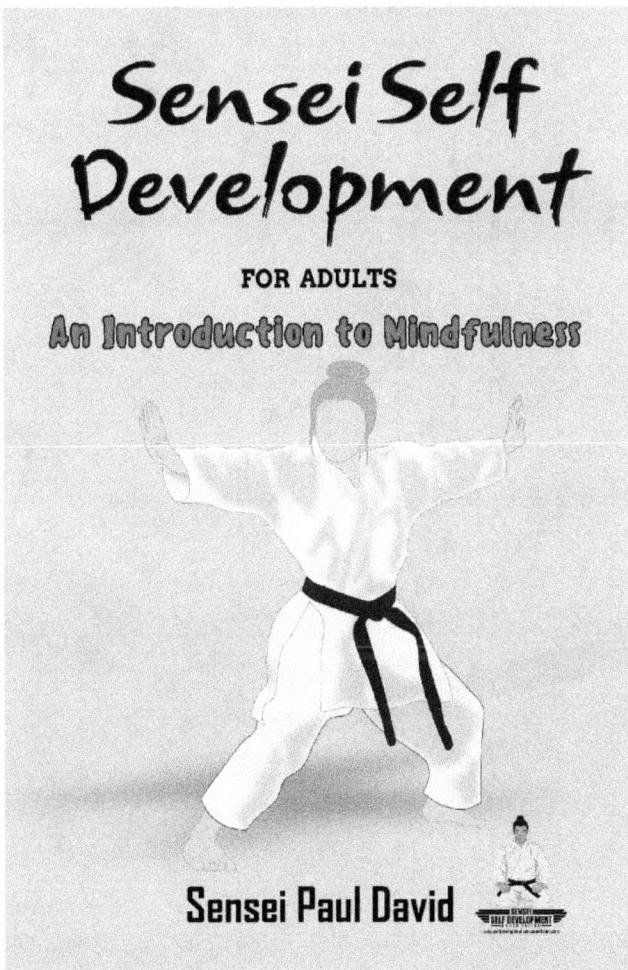

Sensei Self Development

FOR ADULTS

An Introduction to Mindfulness

Sensei Paul David

Check Out The SSD Chronicles Series CLICK HERE

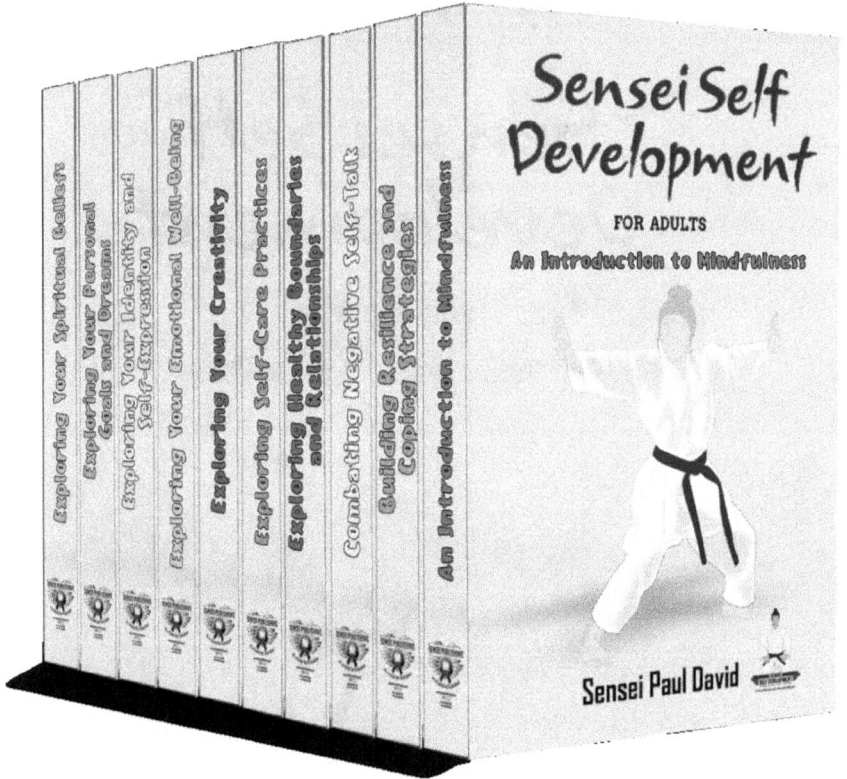

Exploring Your Spiritual Beliefs

Exploring Your Personal Goals and Dreams

Exploring Your Identity and Self-Expression

Exploring Your Emotional Well-Being

Exploring Your Creativity

Exploring Self-Care Practices

Exploring Healthy Boundaries and Relationships

Combating Negative Self-Talk

Building Resilience and Coping Strategies

An Introduction to Mindfulness

Sensei Self Development

FOR ADULTS

An Introduction to Mindfulness

Sensei Paul David

Dedication

To those who courageously take action towards self-improvement - you are helping to evolve the world for generations to come.

- It's a great day to be alive!

If Found Please Contact:

_____

Reward If Found:

_____

MY
COMMITMENT

I, _____

commit to writing This Sensei Self Development Journal for at least 10 days in a row, starting: _____

Writing this journal is valuable to me because:

_____

_____

_____

_____

_____

_____

If I finish a minimum of 10 consecutive days of writing in this journal, I will reward myself by:

_____

_____

_____

_____

_____

_____

If I don't finish 10 days of writing this journal, I will promise to:

_____

_____

_____

_____

_____

I will do the following things to ensure that I write in my Sensei Self Development Journal every day:

_____

_____

_____

_____

_____

Get/Share Your FREE All-Ages Mental Health eBook Now at

www.senseiselfdevelopment.com

Or CLICK HERE

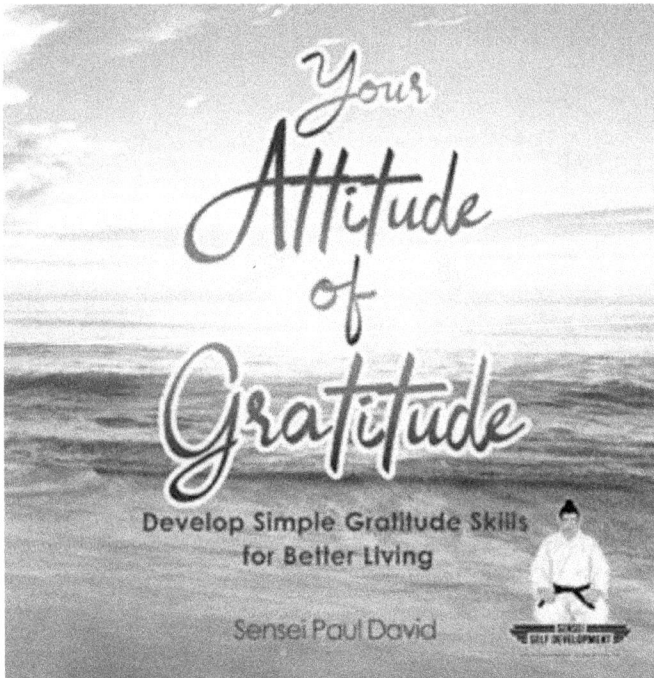

senseiselfdevelopment.com

Check Out Another Book In The
SSD BOOK SERIES:

senseipublishing.com/SSD_SERIES

CLICK HERE

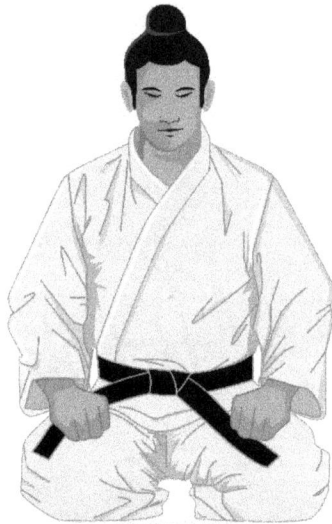

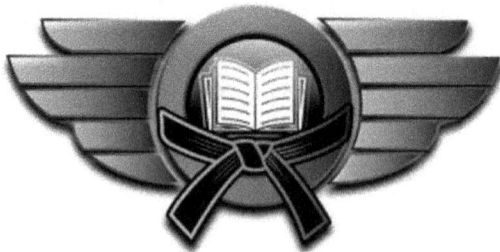

Join Our Publishing Journey!

If you would like to receive FUTURE FREE BOOKS and get to know us better, please click www.senseipublishing.com and join our newsletter by entering your email address in the pop-up box.

Follow Our Blog: senseipauldavid.ca

Follow/Like/Subscribe: Facebook, Instagram, YouTube: @senseipublishing

Scan the QR Code with your phone or tablet

to follow us on social media: Like / Subscribe / Follow

A Message From The Author:
Sensei Paul David

Dear Reader,

Welcome to the world of mental health journaling – a sacred space for self-reflection, growth, and healing. Within these pages, you hold the power to uplift your spirit, invigorate your mind, and nourish your goals.

In a world that often moves at blink-and-you'll-miss-it speed, it's crucial to make time for self-care and self-discovery.

Anxiety, stress, and emotional turbulence may have clouded your mind, making it difficult to find clarity and peace within. But fear not! Together, we will navigate the labyrinth of emotions, and experiences, helping to simplify the path to mental well-being.

This journal is not merely a bunch of blank pages awaiting your words. It is your compassionate companion, offering solace and understanding during your unique journey. Here, you are free to unburden yourself, celebrate small and large victories, and confront the challenges that may still linger.

Within the sheltered realm of these pages, there is no judgment, no expectation, and no pressure. Your unique experience and perspective hold immeasurable worth, and your voice deserves to be heard. Whether you choose to fill the lines with eloquence or simply scribble fragments of your thoughts, please remember each entry is a valuable contribution to your growth.

In this sacred space, you are challenged to take off the mask we so often wear in the outside world. It is here that you can be raw, vulnerable, and authentic – allowing your true self to be seen and embraced without reservation. By giving yourself permission to explore the depths of your emotions and confront the shadows that may lurk within, you will discover profound insights and find the healing you seek over time.

As you embark on this journaling journey, I encourage you to embrace the process itself rather than fixate solely on the outcome. Remember, it is not about reaching a certain destination or ticking off boxes on a list of accomplishments. Rather, it is about cultivating self-awareness, fostering self-compassion, and nurturing a sense of curiosity about the intricate workings of your intelligently beautiful mind.

In the quiet moments of reflection, let your pen become a bridge between your inner world and the possibilities that lie ahead. Create a sanctuary for your thoughts, fears, triumphs, and dreams. As you pour your heart onto these pages, allow your words to be a living testament to courage, resilience, and an unwavering commitment to your own well-being.

I am honored to be a part of your journey, and I believe in your ability to navigate the twists and turns with grace and resilience. Remember, you are not alone in this – countless others have walked similar paths, faced similar challenges, and emerged stronger and wiser on the other side. You have the power to reclaim all of your untapped joy, cultivate a positive mindset that serves you, and foster a deep sense of self-love and peaceful confident. – And it will take a worth effort and time.

So, open the first page of this journal with hope, curiosity, and an open heart and open mind. Embrace the transformative power of self-reflection, and allow it to guide you towards a life of greater fulfilment and peace. Each journaling session is an opportunity to not only connect with yourself but also to rekindle the light within that sometimes flickers but never extinguishes.

Remember, the pages you are about to fill are not just a record of your journey but also a testament to your strength, resilience, and indomitable spirit. Cherish this space, invest in yourself, and let your words be an ode to the magnificent journey of becoming whole.

With great respect for your decision to evolve,

Paul

MY CONVICTION

Please circle your answers below

I am DECIDING to be patient with myself and this PROCESS each time I journal toward my improved state of mental well-being

YES   NO

"The present moment is filled with joy and happiness. If you are attentive, you will see it."

Thich Nhat Hanh

Introduction

The term "art" often carries an air of highbrow exclusivity, conjuring images of mandatory novel readings, museum visits, or films lacking blockbuster thrills. But at its core, art is simply the infusion of our everyday existence with creativity. It's this creative spark that transforms the mundane into the extraordinary, filling us with vitality and joy.

Yet, if we define art as life enriched by creativity, aren't we just cloaking one mystery with another? What, after all, is creativity?

To demystify this, consider these five truths about creativity:

1. Creativity creates something new

Changing our words, for instance, can change how we see things. For instance, long ago, a road was just a path, and the ocean, a vast, intimidating blue. But in "Beowulf," the poet called the ocean a "whale-road," and suddenly, it seemed different. To us, the ocean is a barrier, but to whales, it's a wide-open road.

The phrase was able to create a way of percieving that was never imagined before

2. Creativity Hides

Creativity is an elusive artist, often working unseen. Its magic lies in presenting the novel as if it were always there. The term "whale-road" seamlessly combines two familiar words, unveiling a new vision of the ocean that feels intuitively right, as if waiting to be discovered. Creativity doesn't just solve problems; it uncovers them. It was not known that our language for the ocean was lacking until "whale-road" was coined, and suddenly, it made perfect sense. Creativity excels in this self-effacement.

This concept is crucial in understanding scientific creativity too. We often view science as a series of definitive truths about the world. But isn't scientific discovery also a form of creativity? Consider Newton's second law of motion: it was a creative revelation as profound as "whale-road." Newton's insight, like the poetic metaphor, appeared to describe something always true, yet previously unarticulated. The more successful the creative act, the more it seems like it was always a part of our reality. Creativity, thus, is a master of disguise.

3. Creativity as Life's Essence

Creativity isn't just an occasional spark; it's a constant flow, permeating every facet of existence. It's like the ocean's water filling a sandcastle, shaping and defining the spaces between our moments, actions, and words. This pervasive nature of creativity means you can be inventive in almost anything – the way you walk, cope with grief, build friendships, stretch in the morning, or hum a tune. Our lives are an ongoing canvas of creativity; it's what makes life vibrant and possible, just as water holds a sandcastle together. A life devoid of creativity is like a dry, crumbling structure.

4. The Heartbreak of Creativity

Creativity is not without its risks – it's a venture that can lead to heartache. People often ask why creativity isn't more widespread, why there's imitation or adherence to formulas in art. The reason is simple: creativity can fail. The risk of failure, of looking and feeling foolish, is inherent in creative endeavors. It's this vulnerability that makes creativity both exhilarating and daunting. Just like love, creativity involves the risk of pain and failure, but it's also where its greatest joys are found.

5. Creativity as a Form of Love

The connection between creativity and love is profound. Both involve seeing and making the world anew. Creativity, like love, can be transformative and life-affirming, yet it shares the same fragility and fear of misinterpretation. We guard our creative and loving selves, wary of misrepresentation or manipulation.

Just as we resist reductive explanations of our affections, we protect our creative impulses from being diminished or exploited. The phrase 'corruptio optimi pessima' (the corruption of the best is the worst) aptly captures this sentiment. Love, the most enriching aspect of our existence, when misused or misunderstood, can lead to the deepest despair. Creativity, in its purest form, is akin to love – capable of infusing life with unparalleled beauty and meaning, yet equally susceptible to misinterpretation and misuse.

Fast Facts

Creativity as a Learned Skill: The idea of the 'born genius' is just a myth. Creativity is like a muscle that grows stronger with practice, experimentation, and continuous learning.

Good for Mental Health: Getting creative is not just fun, it's healing. It helps reduce stress, depression, and anxiety, leading to a happier, more balanced mind.

Failure is Part of the Process: Remember, every mistake is a lesson. Being creative means trying, failing, and learning. That's how great ideas are born.

Brain Flexibility and Creativity: Our brains can adapt and change, forming new connections – vital for creative thinking. Learning new things and seeking new experiences keep our creative juices flowing.

Creativity Boost from Sleep: Ever wonder why you get great ideas after a good night's sleep? REM sleep enhances creative problem-solving by letting our brains make unique connections.

Exercise to Spark Creativity: Regular physical activity does more than keep you fit; it boosts your brainpower. Exercise increases blood flow to the brain, making you feel more energetic and ready to think creatively.

Ambient Noise and Creativity: A bit of background noise, like the buzz of a café, can actually help your creativity. It promotes abstract thinking, which is key for coming up with new ideas.

Daydreaming is Useful: Letting your mind wander isn't a waste of time. It can lead to increased creativity, helping your brain make new connections and come up with fresh ideas.

Creativity at Different Times: We're often more creative when we're not at our peak. Early birds might get their best ideas in the morning, and night owls could be more creative at night.

Change of Scenery Helps: Sometimes, just changing where you work can spark new ideas. Different environments stimulate new thoughts and perspectives.

Multitasking is Bad: Juggling too many things at once can actually dampen creativity. It keeps your brain too busy with switching tasks to think creatively.

Breaks for Better Ideas: Taking regular breaks, especially after focusing hard, helps keep creativity high. It gives your brain time to rest and form new ideas.

How to Explore Your Creativity

1. By tuning in to sources of creativity

Creativity surrounds us; it's a matter of tuning into it.

Our creative sources stem from everything we encounter: what we see, do, think, feel, imagine, forget, and even the unspoken or unthought elements within us. These myriad experiences serve as our creative building blocks. This material doesn't come from within us; it's sourced from a wisdom that envelops us, an endless reservoir always accessible. We connect with it through sensing, remembering, or tuning in. It's not limited to our experiences but includes dreams, intuitions, subliminal fragments, and other undiscovered ways the external world infiltrates our inner psyche. To our minds, this material seems to originate internally, but that's an illusion. It's actually fragments of a vast external source within us. These fragments rise from our unconscious like vapor, forming thoughts and ideas.

We act as antennas for creative thought, with some signals stronger than others. If our antenna isn't finely tuned, we might miss the subtler, more valuable messages amidst the noise. These signals are more energetic than tactile, perceived intuitively rather than consciously.

Mostly, we gather data through our five senses. But with higher frequency information, we're channeling energy that can't be physically captured. This energy is illogical, much like an electron being in two places at once. It's immensely valuable, yet few are open enough to receive it.

To detect this indescribable, inaudible signal, we don't actively search or analyze. We create an open space for it, free from the clutter of our usual thoughts, acting as a vacuum to draw down the universe's ideas.

Achieving this openness isn't as hard as it seems. We all start with it. As children, we effortlessly absorbed ideas, delighted by new information without prejudice or comparison. We lived in the moment, spontaneous and curious, experiencing wonder and rapidly shifting emotions without pretense or attachment to narratives.

Artists who continually produce great works often maintain these childlike traits. Embracing a way of being that views the world with uncorrupted, innocent eyes allows you to synchronize with the universe's rhythm.

One effective practice to enhance creativity is the "Daily Inspiration Walk." This simple, yet powerful exercise involves taking a short walk each day, ideally in a natural setting or a place that inspires you. During the walk, consciously engage all your senses to absorb the environment around you. Notice the colors, sounds, textures, smells, and even the taste of the air. Observe people, animals, plants, and inanimate objects with curiosity.

Carry a small notebook or use a voice recording app on your phone. Whenever something catches your attention or sparks a thought, jot it down or record it. It could be anything from the pattern of leaves on a tree, the rhythm of your footsteps, to an overheard snippet of conversation.

After your walk, set aside some time to reflect on your observations. Look for patterns, connections, or contrasts in what you noted. Use these reflections as a springboard for creative work, whether it's writing, drawing, composing music, or brainstorming ideas for a project.

This practice not only hones your observational skills but also helps in developing a habit of seeing the extraordinary in the ordinary, a key aspect of creativity. It encourages you to find inspiration in everyday surroundings, reminding you that sources of creativity are all around, waiting to be discovered.

Looking for Hints

Everywhere we turn, we are surrounded by potential inspiration for our creative endeavors. It's interwoven in our daily conversations, the natural world, chance meetings, and existing artistic creations. When searching for a solution to a creative challenge, be observant of your surroundings. Look for hints that might suggest novel approaches or ways to enhance current concepts.

For instance, a writer in a café, struggling with a character's dialogue, might overhear a snippet of conversation that sparks the perfect response or at least hints at a new direction. We often encounter such guiding messages, provided we stay receptive to them. These insights could jump out at us from a book, a line in a movie might compel us to pause and reflect. Sometimes, they offer the precise solution we seek. Or they might echo a recurring thought, urging us to pay more attention or confirming our current course.

These messages are subtle and omnipresent, yet easily overlooked if we're not actively searching for them. Recognizing connections and contemplating their significance is crucial. When something unusual occurs, question its deeper implications. This pursuit is more an art than a science. We can't force these insights to appear, nor can we always predict their arrival. At times, a clear intention to find an answer or confirmation may help. Other times, releasing all intentions opens new paths.

For artists, interpreting these signals is a fundamental part of the creative process. The more receptive you are, the more effortlessly these insights will come to you. You might start to rely less on rational thought and more on intuitive understanding.

Many people have had ideas this way. J.K. Rowling, for instance, has mentioned that the idea for the Harry Potter series came to her during a delayed train journey. She suddenly had the idea of a young boy attending a school of wizardry. She didn't have a pen and was too shy to ask for one, so she spent the next four hours thinking about the idea, which eventually turned into the Harry Potter series.

Here's how Slinky was invented: Richard James, a naval engineer, was working with springs to support and stabilize sensitive instruments aboard ships. One day, a spring fell off a shelf and continued moving. This inspired the idea for the Slinky, a toy that "walks" down steps.

All in all, be open to associate two dissimilar things together. Look at the idea of Santa Claus. It's the idea of flight combined with a sledge and friendly old man. All of these ideas came together and made a religious tradition over the years.

So allow your mind to freely associate ideas.

Consume Great Works

Immerse yourself in a diverse array of exceptional works. This could involve exploring renowned literature, iconic films, significant artworks, and architectural marvels. Greatness in art is subjective and ever-evolving, varying across different cultures and times. By exposing ourselves to these varied expressions of human creativity, we open ourselves to new perspectives and ideas.

If, for instance, you choose to read classic literature every day for a year instead of following the news, your sensitivity to the nuances of greatness in literature will be more finely honed compared to what you might glean from media. This principle applies to all choices: the friends we keep, the conversations we engage in, and even the thoughts we ponder. These elements influence our ability to discern good from very good, and very good from great, guiding us in what deserves our time and attention.

Given the endless amount of information available and our limited capacity to process it, we might consider carefully curating the quality of what we permit into our lives. This is not just relevant for aspiring artists. For example, even if your aim is to create fast food, the end product will likely be better if you indulge in high-quality fast food during its creation. The goal is to refine our internal gauge of greatness, to inform the myriad choices that could lead to our own significant contributions.

Look at Nature

Among all the profound experiences available to us, nature stands as the most absolute and enduring. It offers a panorama of change across seasons, visible in the mountains, oceans, deserts, and forests. We observe the nightly dance of the moon and stars, finding endless awe and inspiration in the great outdoors. Imagine devoting our lives to observing the subtle shifts of light and shadow through the day; we would continually uncover new wonders.

Appreciating nature doesn't require understanding it, a truth that applies to all beautiful things. It's about being present in moments that take our breath away, whether it's watching a line of birds weave through a dimming sky or standing in awe at the base of an ancient redwood. Nature is rich with wisdom, sparking possibilities within us and bringing us closer to our own essence.

Consider the act of choosing colors: a Pantone book offers a limited range, but nature presents an infinite palette. Every rock displays a myriad of hues, each so unique that no paint can perfectly replicate it. Nature defies our attempts to categorize and simplify. It is far richer, more interconnected, and complex than we often realize – a world filled with mystery and beauty.

Deepening our connection with nature not only nourishes our spirit but also enriches our artistic expression. The closer we align with the natural world, the more we understand our unity with it.

Look Inward

A breeze, seemingly cool yet simultaneously warm, brushes against my skin, causing a shiver. With eyes shut, I hear the harmonious melody of a distant stream. Closer, a trio of birds engages in an unplanned chorus, their location just behind and to my left. The smallest bird, its chirp sharp and quick, adds a distinct layer to the natural symphony. The birds, each with their own rhythm, create a tapestry of sound that feels more like parallel solos than a conversation.

The world around me contributes its own notes: the faint laughter of children in the distance, the rhythm of a distant drummer, a soft murmur of conversation nearby. An occasional itch tingles on my right cheek, near my jawline. Then, the deep hum of a nearby car passing by briefly overlays a snippet of classical music, a tune I vaguely remember playing softly earlier, now brought to the forefront of my awareness.

As someone approaches, my eyes flutter open, and the vividness of this auditory and sensory world fades, replaced by the immediate reality.

Many people view life as a sequence of external events, believing that only an outwardly remarkable life is worth sharing. However, this perspective often leads to neglecting the richness of our internal experiences.

By turning our attention inward — to our feelings, sensations, and the flow of our thoughts — we uncover a treasure trove of content. Our inner world is as fascinating, beautiful, and unexpected as nature itself, stemming from the same origin. In exploring our internal landscape, we process and connect with the external world, realizing that these aspects are not separate but intertwined.

Both a striking thought and a breathtaking sunset are equally beautiful.

Recognizing this broadens our perspective, revealing a plethora of experiences that are more diverse and profound than we might initially perceive.

Step Away (or Distract Yourself)

Distraction, when skillfully employed, is an invaluable tool for artists. It can be essential in navigating the creative process. Consider meditation: as the mind begins to quiet, it often encounters interruptions like worries or random thoughts. To counter this, many meditation practices introduce a mantra. This repetitive phrase occupies the conscious mind, preventing disruptive thoughts and thereby acting as a form of distraction.

Similarly, objects like worry beads, rosaries, and malas serve to engage the conscious mind, allowing the subconscious to work more freely. In creative endeavors, hitting a roadblock often necessitates stepping away from the work at hand. By keeping the problem in the background of our thoughts and engaging in simple, routine activities — such as driving, walking, swimming, or even washing dishes — we create mental space for solutions to emerge.

Physical movement can also be a catalyst for creativity. Some musicians, for instance, find that they compose melodies more effectively while driving than when sitting in a studio. These distractions occupy one part of the mind, liberating the rest for creative thinking. This process might tap into different brain areas, offering new perspectives that the direct approach might miss.

It's important to differentiate distraction from procrastination. Procrastination hinders productivity, while strategic distraction serves the creative process. It's not about avoiding work but redirecting our focus in a way that facilitates creativity.

Cultivating Patience

Patience is a crucial ingredient in the creative process. It's essential for absorbing information accurately and for creating work that deeply resonates, embodying all we wish to express. Every aspect of an artist's work and life stands to benefit from the cultivation of this attainable habit.

Much like awareness, patience is developed through accepting the present moment as it is. Impatience, on the other hand, is essentially a resistance to reality. It manifests as a desire for things to be different – for time to move faster, for tomorrow to arrive sooner, or for a wishful leap to another place or time. However, since time is beyond our control, patience begins with embracing natural rhythms and processes.

Ironically, the perceived advantage of impatience – to save time by hastening and bypassing these rhythms – often ends up consuming more time and energy, resulting in wasted effort.

In creativity, patience means accepting that much of the creative process is not under our direct control. We can't force greatness; our role is to invite it and wait actively, but not anxiously, as anxiety can repel the very inspiration we seek. Patience involves a continuous, open-hearted readiness.

If we remove the pressure of time from a work's development, we're left with pure patience. This applies not just to the creation of the work itself, but to the ongoing growth of the artist.

Even those masterpieces produced under tight deadlines are the culmination of years, sometimes decades, of patient work on other projects. In the world of creativity, the constant need for patience is perhaps one of the most unyielding rules.

Don't Wait for Inspiration to Strike

The journey of an artist is not merely a waiting game for inspiration. While inspiration can be elusive and beyond our control, active effort is within our control. In its absence, we can still progress by focusing on different aspects of our projects, independent of that elusive creative spark.

Regular commitment to your craft is crucial. To stimulate inspiration, try altering your inputs. Watch a movie without sound, listen to the same song repeatedly, read only the first word of each sentence in a story, sort stones by size or color, or explore lucid dreaming. Break your routines, seek out differences, and draw connections.

Awe is a key sign of inspiration. We often overlook the marvels of nature and human invention that surround us. How do we move beyond disconnection and numbness to appreciate the wonders of our world? Most things can inspire awe if viewed with fresh eyes. Train yourself to see the extraordinary in the ordinary. Immerse yourself in this perspective as much as possible. The beauty in the world not only enriches our lives but also sets a standard for our work. Strive to develop an eye for harmony and balance, crafting your creations as if they were natural elements of the world, timeless and essential, like mountains or feathers.

Practice Your Craft

If you never practice your craft, you can never create a work of art. You cannot expect to come up with a movie if you don't know the structure of screenplays. You cannot write poetry if you are unfamiliar with rhythm. You cannot devise the theory of gravitation without knowledge in mathematics and physics.

Newton, often depicted as merely a curious individual, was in fact exceptional in physics and mathematics. This exemplifies why it's rare to find a 10 or 15-year-old who has truly created something unique. If creativity is so abundant in children, why don't they produce groundbreaking work? The answer lies in their lack of mastery over their craft.

In "Age and Great Invention," Benjamin Jones, a researcher at the National Bureau of Economic Research, analyzed data on Nobel Prize winners in Physics, Chemistry, Medicine, and Economics over a century, along with major technological innovations during that time.

His findings revealed a compelling pattern: no significant achievements were produced by innovators before the age of 19, and only 7 percent were achieved by those at or before the age of 26 (which was Einstein's age during his groundbreaking work).

This suggests that while innate talent is important, it's the honing of one's skills and knowledge over years of dedicated practice that truly leads to exceptional creativity and innovation. Thus, creativity is important, but it practice to access it to reveal its full potential.

This is non-negotiable.

Before We Get Started…

Remember, mindfulness journaling is a personal practice, and these questions are meant to guide and inspire you. Feel free to adapt and modify them to suit your needs and preferences. Explore, reflect, and embrace the opportunity to deepen your self-awareness and cultivate a sense of inner peace.

Date ___ / ___ / ___ : S M T W Th F S

I feel: 😊 😁 😋 😞 😠
(please circle) because because because because because
_____ _____ _____ _____ _____
_____ _____ _____ _____ _____

Today I Am Grateful For

1. _____
2. _____
3. _____

What could help transform today into a remarkable day?

Reflective Writing

What is the most creative project you have
undertaken recently?

_____

_____

_____

_____

_____

_____

_____

Which of these is NOT a way to spark your creativity?

A) Taking a walk in nature
B) Doing the same routine every day
C) Trying a new hobby
D) Listening to music

All Are Correct - Choose The Response You Feel Is Most Important To Remember

Date ___ / ___ / ___ : S M T W Th F S

I feel:
(please circle)

because because because because because

_____ _____ _____ _____ _____
_____ _____ _____ _____ _____

Today I Am Grateful For

1. _____
2. _____
3. _____

What could help transform today into a remarkable day?

Reflective Writing

What was the biggest challenge you faced when engaging in creative endeavors?

_____

_____

_____

_____

_____

_____

_____

Which of these is a common barrier to creativity?

A) Fear of failure
B) Lack of motivation
C) Too much sleep
D) Too many ideas

All Are Correct - Choose The Response You Feel Is Most Important To Remember

Date ___ / ___ / ___: S M T W Th F S

I feel:
(please circle)

because _____ because _____ because _____ because _____ because _____

Today I Am Grateful For

1. _____
2. _____
3. _____

What could help transform today into a remarkable day?

Reflective Writing

What do you do to keep your creativity flowing?

_____

_____

_____

_____

_____

_____

_____

_____

What can you do to overcome a creative block?

A) Keep pushing through until you come up with something
B) Take a break and do a different activity
C) Give up and try again the next day
D) Wait for inspiration to strike

All Are Correct - Choose The Response You Feel Is Most Important To Remember

Date ___ / ___ / ___: S M T W Th F S

I feel: 😊 😁 😋 😣 😠
(please circle) because because because because because
_____ _____ _____ _____ _____
_____ _____ _____ _____ _____

Today I Am Grateful For

1. _____
2. _____
3. _____

What could help transform today into a remarkable day?

Reflective Writing

How have you learned to overcome creative blocks?

_____

_____

_____

_____

_____

_____

_____

Which of these is NOT a type of creativity?

A) Visual

B) Musical

C) Athletic

D) Linguistic

All Are Correct - Choose The Response You Feel Is Most Important To Remember

Date ___ / ___ / ___ : S   M   T   W   Th   F   S

I feel:
(please circle)

because   because   because   because   because
_____   _____   _____   _____   _____
_____   _____   _____   _____   _____

Today I Am Grateful For

1. _____
2. _____
3. _____

What could help transform today into a remarkable day?

Reflective Writing

What have been some of the successes you have experienced when being creative?

_____

_____

_____

_____

_____

_____

_____

How does setting a deadline help with creativity?

A) It adds pressure and can spark new ideas
B) It allows for more time to think and plan
C) It restricts creativity and limits ideas
D) It makes the end result less important

All Are Correct - Choose The Response You Feel Is Most Important To Remember

Date ___ / ___ / ___ : S   M   T   W   Th   F   S

I feel:
(please circle)

because   because   because   because   because
_____   _____   _____   _____   _____
_____   _____   _____   _____   _____

Today I Am Grateful For

1. _____
2. _____
3. _____

What could help transform today into a remarkable day?

Reflective Writing

What is your favorite creative outlet?

_____

_____

_____

_____

_____

_____

_____

_____

Which of these is NOT a characteristic of a creative person?

A) High levels of self-doubt

B) Curiosity and open-mindedness

C) Ability to think outside the box

D) Flexibility and adaptability

All Are Correct - Choose The Response You Feel Is Most Important To Remember

Date ___ / ___ / ___ : S   M   T   W   Th   F   S

I feel:
(please circle)

because _____ because _____ because _____ because _____ because _____

Today I Am Grateful For

1. _____
2. _____
3. _____

What could help transform today into a remarkable day?

Reflective Writing

How has exploring your creativity impacted your life?

_____

_____

_____

_____

_____

_____

_____

_____

How can collaboration with others enhance creativity?

A) It allows for a diversity of perspectives and ideas
B) It limits individual creativity and originality
C) It creates competition and rivalry
D) It adds pressure and stress

All Are Correct - Choose The Response You Feel Is Most Important To Remember

41

Date ___ / ___ / ___ : S   M   T   W   Th   F   S

I feel:
(please circle)

because _____ because _____ because _____ because _____ because _____

Today I Am Grateful For

1. _____
2. _____
3. _____

What could help transform today into a remarkable day?

Reflective Writing

How do you handle creative criticism?

_____
_____
_____
_____
_____
_____
_____
_____
_____

Which of these is a common misconception about creativity?

A) It's only for artists and musicians
B) It can't be learned or improved
C) It requires constant inspiration and motivation
D) It's a fixed trait and cannot change

All Are Correct - Choose The Response You Feel Is Most Important To Remember

Date ___ / ___ / ___ : S   M   T   W   Th   F   S

I feel:
(please circle)

because _____ because _____ because _____ because _____ because _____

Today I Am Grateful For

1. _____
2. _____
3. _____

What could help transform today into a remarkable day?

Reflective Writing

What are some of the most creative ideas you have had?

_____

_____

_____

_____

_____

_____

_____

How can keeping a journal or sketchbook help with creativity?

A) It provides a space to record and reflect on ideas
B) It takes up too much time and energy
C) It limits creativity to just writing or drawing
D) It's only for professionals, not amateurs

All Are Correct - Choose The Response You Feel Is Most Important To Remember

Date ___ / ___ / ___: S M T W Th F S

I feel:
(please circle)

because _____ because _____ because _____ because _____ because _____

Today I Am Grateful For

1. _____
2. _____
3. _____

What could help transform today into a remarkable day?

Reflective Writing

How has exploring your creativity enabled you to become a better problem solver?

_____

_____

_____

_____

_____

_____

_____

Which of these is NOT a way to foster a creativity-friendly environment?

A) Surrounding yourself with clutter and disorganization
B) Removing distractions such as social media or TV
C) Having a designated creative space
D) Surrounding yourself with art and inspirational quotes

All Are Correct - Choose The Response You Feel Is Most Important To Remember

Date ___ / ___ / ___ : S   M   T   W   Th   F   S

I **feel:**
(please circle)

because   because   because   because   because
_____   _____   _____   _____   _____
_____   _____   _____   _____   _____

Today I Am Grateful For

1. _____
2. _____
3. _____

What could help transform today into a remarkable day?

Reflective Writing

What do you do when you feel stuck in a creative rut?

_____

_____

_____

_____

_____

_____

_____

How can taking risks and being vulnerable enhance creativity?

A) It leads to more failures and setbacks
B) It allows for experimentation and new ideas
C) It leads to decreased confidence and motivation
D) It limits creativity to safe and comfortable choices

All Are Correct - Choose The Response You Feel Is Most Important To Remember

Date ___/___/___: S M T W Th F S

I feel:
(please circle)

because because because because because

_____ _____ _____ _____ _____
_____ _____ _____ _____ _____

Today I Am Grateful For

1. _____
2. _____
3. _____

What could help transform today into a remarkable day?

Reflective Writing
How do you go about generating new and innovative ideas?

_____

_____

_____

_____

_____

_____

_____

_____

Which of these is NOT a way to incorporate playfulness into creativity?

A) Taking things too seriously and avoiding mistakes

B) Trying new things and being open to failure

C) Engaging in activities without a specific goal or outcome

D) Embracing curiosity and imagination

All Are Correct - Choose The Response You Feel Is Most Important To Remember

Date ___ / ___ / ___ : S M T W Th F S

I feel:
(please circle)

because _____ because _____ because _____ because _____ because _____

Today I Am Grateful For

1. _____
2. _____
3. _____

What could help transform today into a remarkable day?

Reflective Writing
What techniques do you use to stay motivated when engaged in creative pursuits?

_____

_____

_____

_____

_____

_____

_____

_____

How can mindfulness and being present help with creativity?

A) It keeps the mind focused and avoids distractions
B) It limits the potential for new ideas and solutions
C) It causes stress and anxiety, hindering creativity
D) It allows for a deeper connection to surroundings and experiences

All Are Correct - Choose The Response You Feel Is Most Important To Remember

Date ___ / ___ / ___: S M T W Th F S

I feel:
(please circle)

because   because   because   because   because
_____ _____ _____ _____ _____
_____ _____ _____ _____ _____

Today I Am Grateful For

1. _____
2. _____
3. _____

What could help transform today into a remarkable day?

Reflective Writing

What tips and tricks have you learned over the
years that help you stay creative?

_____

_____

_____

_____

_____

_____

_____

Which of these is a common misconception about brainstorming?

A) It's just about throwing out random ideas

B) It's only for groups and not for individual creativity

C) It doesn't require any preparation or planning

D) It's ineffective and doesn't lead to innovative solutions

All Are Correct - Choose The Response You Feel Is Most Important To Remember

Date ___ / ___ / ___ : S   M   T   W   Th   F   S

I feel:
(please circle)

because _____   because _____   because _____   because _____   because _____

Today I Am Grateful For

1. _____
2. _____
3. _____

What could help transform today into a remarkable day?

Reflective Writing

What do you feel is the biggest benefit of exploring your creativity?

_____

_____

_____

_____

_____

_____

_____

How can seeking out new experiences and perspectives enhance creativity?

A) It limits creativity to familiar and comfortable ideas
B) It provides inspiration and different ways of thinking
C) It leads to decreased confidence and motivation
D) It doesn't contribute to personal growth or development

All Are Correct - Choose The Response You Feel Is Most Important To Remember

As we reach the final pages of this journey through "Positive Mindset," I want to extend my heartfelt thanks to you. Your commitment to exploring positivity and its transformative power is not only commendable but a testament to your desire for personal growth and a richer, more fulfilling life experience.

Remember, the journey towards a positive mindset is ongoing and ever-evolving. Each day presents new opportunities to apply these principles, to learn, and to grow. I encourage you to revisit these pages whenever you need a reminder of your incredible potential to foster positivity and resilience in the face of life's challenges.

As we part ways, I leave you with a quote that has been a guiding star in my journey: "The greatest discovery of any generation is that a human can alter his life by altering his attitude."

– William James.

Thank you for allowing me to be a part of your journey. May your path be filled with light, hope, and endless possibilities. Farewell, and may you carry the spirit of positivity with you, today and always.

With gratitude and best wishes,

Sensei Paul David

Reflective Writing

_____

_____

_____

_____

_____

_____

_____

_____

_____

_____

_____

_____

_____

_____

_____

_____

_____

_____

_____

_____

_____

_____

_____

The End

As you close the pages of this mindfulness journal, remember that each word you've written is a step on your journey towards self-awareness and inner peace. Embrace the moments of clarity, the revelations, and even the uncertainties you've encountered along the way. Let this journal be a testament to your growth and a reminder that every day offers a new opportunity to be present, to observe, and to appreciate the simple wonders of life. Carry these lessons forward, and may your path be filled with mindful moments and serene reflections. Until we meet again in these pages, be gentle with yourself and stay anchored in the now.

Mindfulness isn't difficult, we just need to remember to do it.

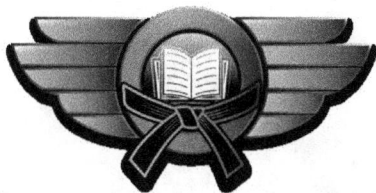

Thank You!

If you found this book helpful, I would be grateful if you would **post an honest review on Amazon** so this book can reach other supportive readers like you!

All you need to do is digitally flip to the back and leave your review. Or visit amazon.com/author/senseipauldavid click the correct book cover and click on the blue link next to the yellow stars that say, "customer reviews."

As always...
It's a great day to be alive!

Get/Share Your FREE SSD Mental Health Chronicles at
www.senseiselfdevelopment.care

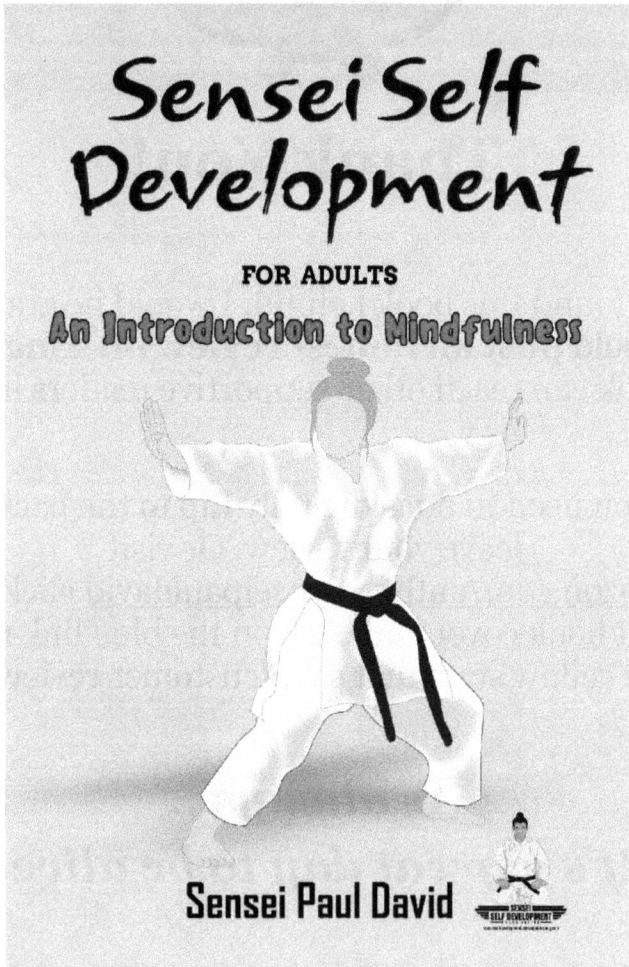

Sensei Self Development

FOR ADULTS

An Introduction to Mindfulness

Sensei Paul David

Check Out The SSD Chronicles Series CLICK HERE

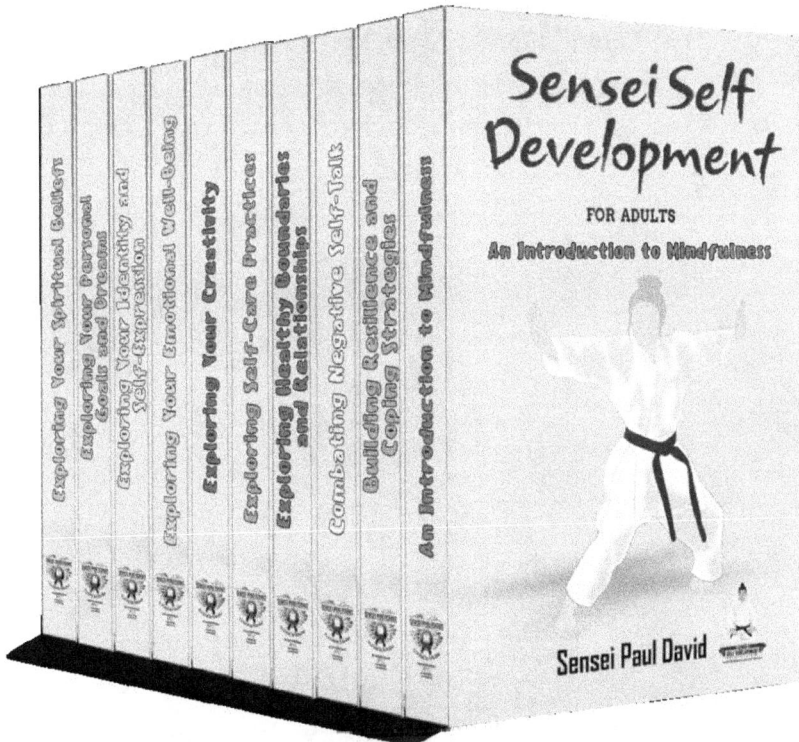

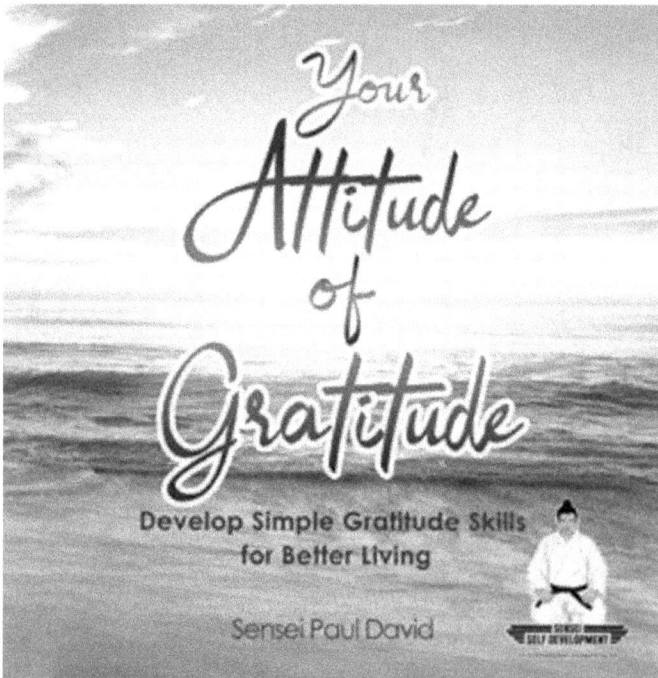

Click Another Book In The SSD BOOK SERIES:

senseipublishing.com/SSD_SERIES

CLICK HERE

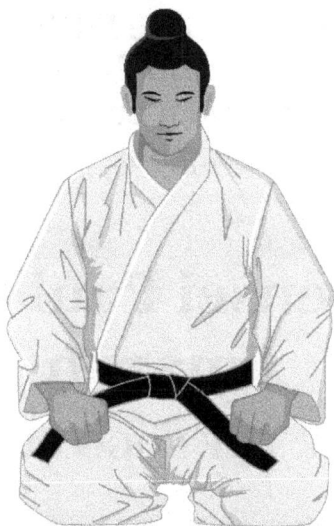

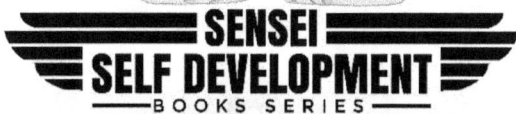

senseiselfdevelopment.senseipublishing.com

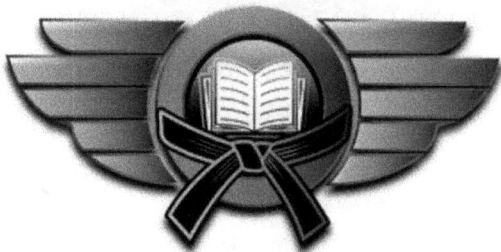

Join Our Publishing Journey!

If you would like to receive FREE BOOKS, please visit **www.senseipublishing.com**. Join our newsletter by entering your email address in the pop-up box

Follow Sensei Paul David on Amazon

CLICK THE LOGO BELOW

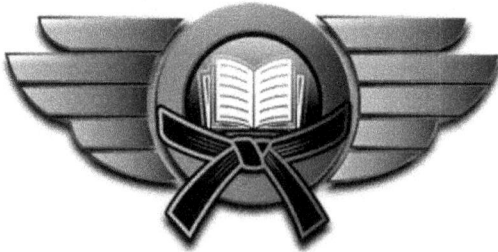

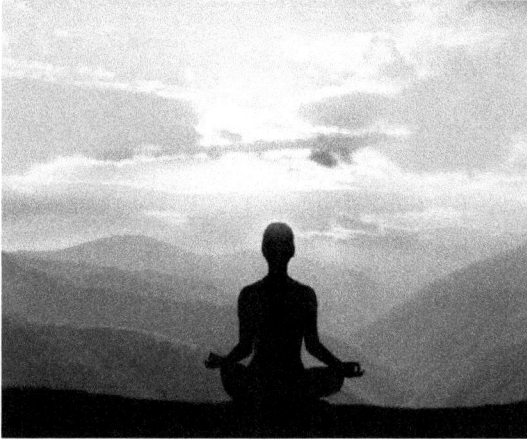

FREE BONUS!!!
Experience Over 25 FREE Engaging Guided Meditations!

Prized Skills & Practices for Adults & Kids. Help Restore Deep-Sleep, Lower Stress, Improve Posture, Navigate Uncertainty & More.

Download the Free Insight Timer App and click the link below:
http://insig.ht/sensei_paul

About Sensei Publishing

Sensei Publishing commits itself to helping people of all ages transform into better versions of themselves by providing high-quality and research-based self-development books with an emphasis on mental health and guided meditations. Sensei Publishing offers well-written e-books, audiobooks, paperbacks and online courses that simplify complicated but practical topics in line with its mission to inspire people towards positive transformation.

It's a great day to be alive!

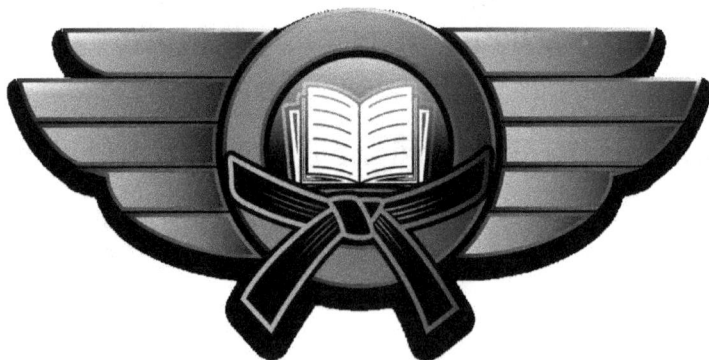

About the Author

I create simple & transformative eBooks & Guided Meditations for Adults & Children proven to help navigate uncertainty, solve niche problems & bring families closer together.

I'm a former finance project manager, private pilot, jiu-jitsu instructor, musician & former University of Toronto Fitness Trainer. I prefer a science-based approach to focus on these & other areas in my life to stay humble & hungry to evolve. I hope you enjoy my work and I'd love to hear your feedback.

- It's a great day to be alive!

Sensei Paul David

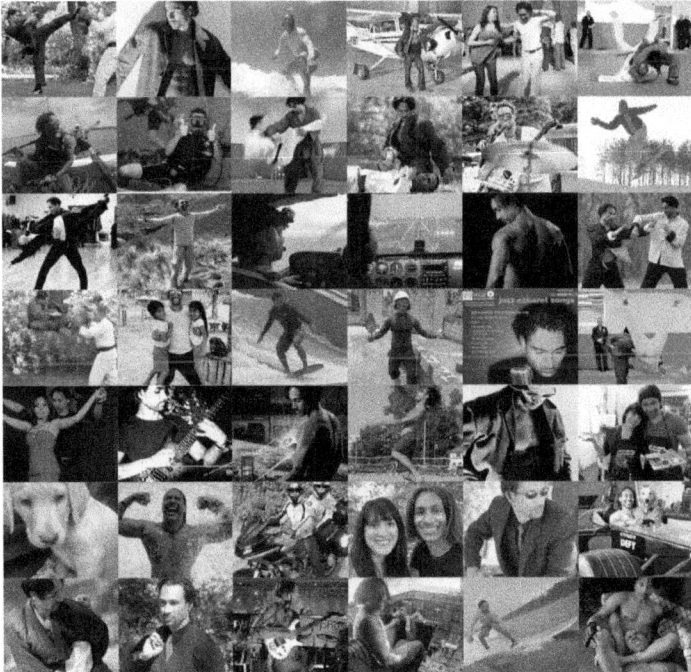

Scan & Follow/Like/Subscribe: Facebook, Instagram,
YouTube: @senseipublishing

Scan using your phone/iPad camera for Social Media
Visit us at www.senseipublishing.com and sign up for our
newsletter to learn more about our exciting books and to
experience our FREE Guided Meditations for Kids & Adults.

www.ingramcontent.com/pod-product-compliance
Lightning Source LLC
Chambersburg PA
CBHW071244020426
42333CB00015B/1614